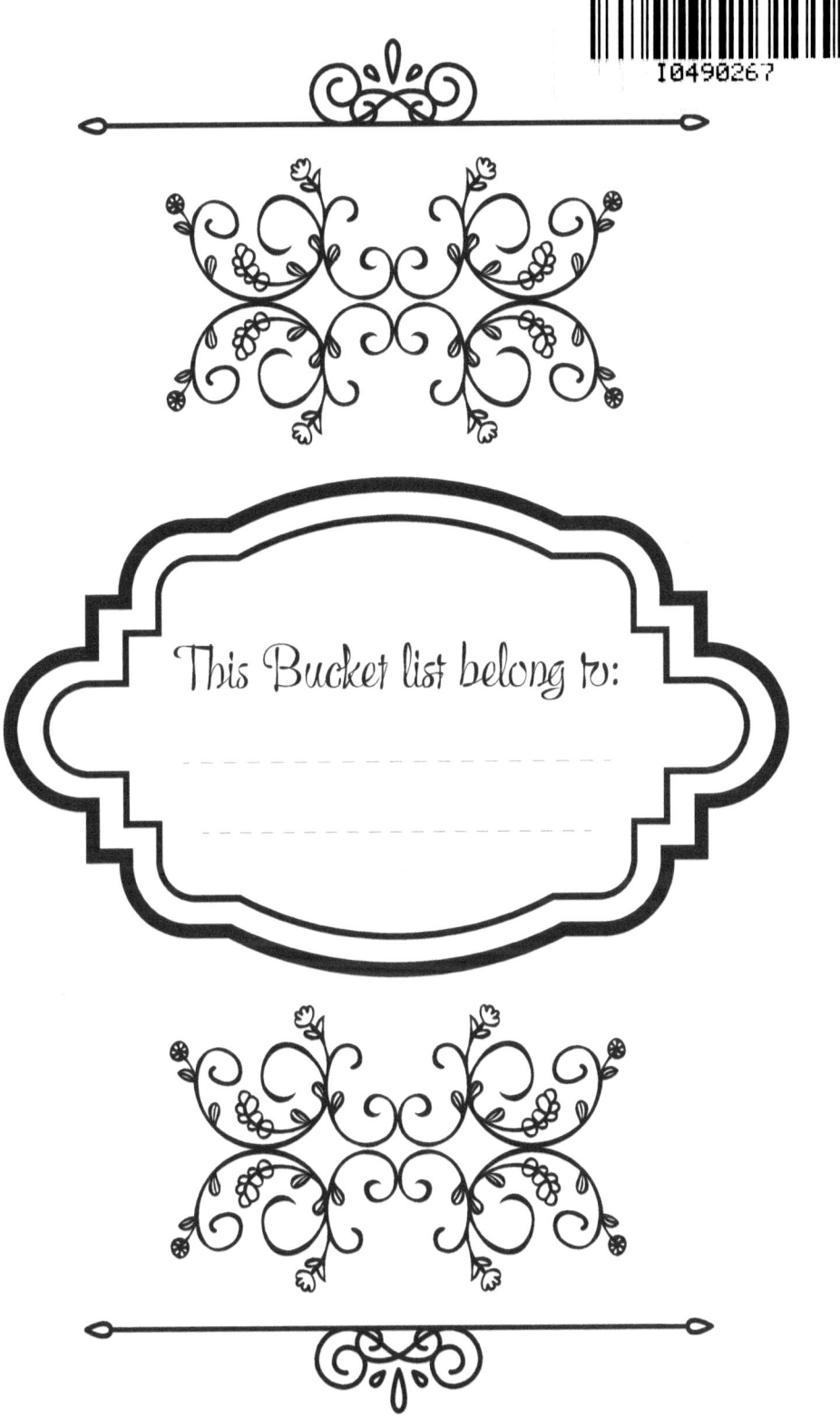

This Bucket list belong to:

My Bucket List Goal ....

....

Date .... Location ....

Reason of doing this:

Actions we have to take:

My Experience:

My Bucket List Goal ---- ---- ---- ----

---- ---- ---- ---- ---- ---- ---- ----

Date ---- ---- ---- Location ---- ---- ---- ----

Reason of doing this:

---- ---- ---- ---- ---- ---- ---- ---- ----

---- ---- ---- ---- ---- ---- ---- ---- ----

---- ---- ---- ---- ---- ---- ---- ---- ----

---- ---- ---- ---- ---- ---- ---- ---- ----

Actions we have to take:

---- ---- ---- ---- ---- ---- ---- ---- ----

---- ---- ---- ---- ---- ---- ---- ---- ----

---- ---- ---- ---- ---- ---- ---- ---- ----

---- ---- ---- ---- ---- ---- ---- ---- ----

---- ---- ---- ---- ---- ---- ---- ---- ----

My Experience:

---- ---- ---- ---- ---- ---- ---- ---- ----

---- ---- ---- ---- ---- ---- ---- ---- ----

---- ---- ---- ---- ---- ---- ---- ---- ----

---- ---- ---- ---- ---- ---- ---- ---- ----

---- ---- ---- ---- ---- ---- ---- ---- ----

My Bucket List Goal ....

....

Date _____ Location _____

Reason of doing this:

Actions we have to take:

My Experience:

My Bucket List Goal ....

....

Date .... Location ....

Reason of doing this:

....

....

....

....

Actions we have to take:

....

....

....

....

....

My Experience:

....

....

....

....

....

My Bucket List Goal _____

_____

Date _____ Location _____

Reason of doing this:

_____
_____
_____
_____

Actions we have to take:

_____
_____
_____
_____
_____
_____

My Experience:

_____
_____
_____
_____
_____

My Bucket List Goal ----------- ------------- ----------- -----------

------------- ------------- ------------- ------------- -------------

Date ------- ------- ------- Location ------- ------- ------- -------

Reason of doing this:

------- ------- ------- ------- ------- ------- ------- ------- -------

------- ------- ------- ------- ------- ------- ------- ------- -------

------- ------- ------- ------- ------- ------- ------- ------- -------

------- ------- ------- ------- ------- ------- ------- ------- -------

Actions we have to take:

------- ------- ------- ------- ------- ------- ------- ------- -------

------- ------- ------- ------- ------- ------- ------- ------- -------

------- ------- ------- ------- ------- ------- ------- ------- -------

------- ------- ------- ------- ------- ------- ------- ------- -------

------- ------- ------- ------- ------- ------- ------- ------- -------

My Experience:

------- ------- ------- ------- ------- ------- ------- ------- -------

------- ------- ------- ------- ------- ------- ------- ------- -------

------- ------- ------- ------- ------- ------- ------- ------- -------

------- ------- ------- ------- ------- ------- ------- ------- -------

My Bucket List Goal

Date _____ Location _____

Reason of doing this:

_____
_____
_____
_____

Actions we have to take:

_____
_____
_____
_____
_____

My Experience:

_____
_____
_____
_____
_____

My Bucket List Goal ....

....

Date .... Location ....

Reason of doing this:

....
....
....
....

Actions we have to take:

....
....
....
....
....

My Experience:

....
....
....
....

My Bucket List Goal _____

_____

Date _____ Location _____

Reason of doing this:

_____
_____
_____
_____

Actions we have to take:

_____
_____
_____
_____
_____

My Experience:

_____
_____
_____
_____
_____

My Bucket List Goal

Date .... Location ....

Reason of doing this:

....
....
....
....

Actions we have to take:

....
....
....
....
....

My Experience:

....
....
....
....
....

My Bucket List Goal

Date _____ Location _____

Reason of doing this:

_____

_____

_____

_____

Actions we have to take:

_____

_____

_____

_____

_____

My Experience:

_____

_____

_____

_____

_____

My Bucket List Goal ----------------------------

Date ---------------- Location ----------------

Reason of doing this:

Actions we have to take:

My Experience:

My Bucket List Goal

Date _____ Location _____

Reason of doing this:

_____

_____

_____

_____

Actions we have to take:

_____

_____

_____

_____

_____

My Experience:

_____

_____

_____

_____

_____

My Bucket List Goal

Date _____   Location _____

Reason of doing this:

_____

_____

_____

_____

Actions we have to take:

_____

_____

_____

_____

_____

_____

My Experience:

_____

_____

_____

_____

_____

My Bucket List Goal _____

_____

Date _____ Location _____

Reason of doing this:

_____
_____
_____
_____

Actions we have to take:

_____
_____
_____
_____
_____
_____

My Experience:

_____
_____
_____
_____
_____

My Bucket List Goal _____

Date _____ Location _____

Reason of doing this:

_____
_____
_____
_____

Actions we have to take:

_____
_____
_____
_____

My Experience:

_____
_____
_____
_____

My Bucket List Goal

Date _____ Location _____

Reason of doing this:

_____

_____

_____

_____

Actions we have to take:

_____

_____

_____

_____

_____

My Experience:

_____

_____

_____

_____

_____

My Bucket List Goal ....

Date .... Location ....

Reason of doing this:

....
....
....
....

Actions we have to take:

....
....
....
....
....
....

My Experience:

....
....
....
....
....
....

My Bucket List Goal

Date _____   Location _____

Reason of doing this:

_____
_____
_____
_____

Actions we have to take:

_____
_____
_____
_____
_____
_____

My Experience:

_____
_____
_____
_____
_____

My Bucket List Goal

Date _____ Location _____

Reason of doing this:

_____
_____
_____
_____

Actions we have to take:

_____
_____
_____
_____
_____

My Experience:

_____
_____
_____
_____
_____

My Bucket List Goal ......

Date .... Location ....

Reason of doing this:
....
....
....
....

Actions we have to take:
....
....
....
....
....

My Experience:
....
....
....
....
....

My Bucket List Goal _____

_____

Date _____ Location _____

Reason of doing this:

Actions we have to take:

My Experience:

My Bucket List Goal

Date _____ Location _____

Reason of doing this:

_____
_____
_____
_____

Actions we have to take:

_____
_____
_____
_____
_____
_____

My Experience:

_____
_____
_____
_____
_____

My Bucket List Goal _____

_____

Date _____ Location _____

Reason of doing this:

Actions we have to take:

My Experience:

My Bucket List Goal _____

_____

Date _____ Location _____

Reason of doing this:

_____

_____

_____

_____

Actions we have to take:

_____

_____

_____

_____

_____

_____

My Experience:

_____

_____

_____

_____

_____

My Bucket List Goal

Date .... Location ....

Reason of doing this:

Actions we have to take:

My Experience:

My Bucket List Goal ....

....

Date .... Location ....

Reason of doing this:

....

....

....

....

Actions we have to take:

....

....

....

....

....

....

My Experience:

....

....

....

....

....

....

My Bucket List Goal _____

_____

Date _____ Location _____

Reason of doing this:

_____
_____
_____
_____

Actions we have to take:

_____
_____
_____
_____
_____
_____

My Experience:

_____
_____
_____
_____
_____
_____

My Bucket List Goal _____

Date _____ Location _____

Reason of doing this:

_____
_____
_____
_____

Actions we have to take:

_____
_____
_____
_____
_____
_____

My Experience:

_____
_____
_____
_____
_____

My Bucket List Goal _____

_____

Date _____ Location _____

Reason of doing this:

_____
_____
_____
_____

Actions we have to take:

_____
_____
_____
_____
_____
_____

My Experience:

_____
_____
_____
_____
_____

My Bucket List Goal _____

_____

Date _____ Location _____

Reason of doing this:

- -
- -
- -
- -

Actions we have to take:

- -
- -
- -
- -
- -

My Experience:

- -
- -
- -
- -
- -

My Bucket List Goal

Date _____ Location _____

Reason of doing this:
_____
_____
_____
_____

Actions we have to take:
_____
_____
_____
_____
_____
_____

My Experience:
_____
_____
_____
_____
_____

My Bucket List Goal _____

_____

Date _____ Location _____

Reason of doing this:

_____
_____
_____
_____

Actions we have to take:

_____
_____
_____
_____
_____
_____

My Experience:

_____
_____
_____
_____
_____

My Bucket List Goal _____

_____

Date _____ Location _____

Reason of doing this:

_____
_____
_____
_____

Actions we have to take:

_____
_____
_____
_____
_____
_____

My Experience:

_____
_____
_____
_____
_____

My Bucket List Goal _____

_____

Date _____ Location _____

Reason of doing this:

_____

_____

_____

_____

Actions we have to take:

_____

_____

_____

_____

_____

_____

My Experience:

_____

_____

_____

_____

_____

My Bucket List Goal _____

_____

Date _____ Location _____

Reason of doing this:

_____

_____

_____

_____

Actions we have to take:

_____

_____

_____

_____

_____

My Experience:

_____

_____

_____

_____

_____

My Bucket List Goal ....

....

Date .... Location ....

Reason of doing this:

....

....

....

....

Actions we have to take:

....

....

....

....

....

....

My Experience:

....

....

....

....

....

My Bucket List Goal

Date _____ Location _____

Reason of doing this:

_____
_____
_____
_____

Actions we have to take:

_____
_____
_____
_____
_____
_____

My Experience:

_____
_____
_____
_____
_____

My Bucket List Goal _____

_____

Date _____ Location _____

Reason of doing this:

_____

_____

_____

_____

Actions we have to take:

_____

_____

_____

_____

_____

_____

My Experience:

_____

_____

_____

_____

_____

My Bucket List Goal ----------------------------

Date ---------------- Location ----------------

Reason of doing this:

Actions we have to take:

My Experience:

My Bucket List Goal

Date _____ Location _____

Reason of doing this:

_____

_____

_____

_____

Actions we have to take:

_____

_____

_____

_____

_____

My Experience:

_____

_____

_____

_____

_____

My Bucket List Goal _____
_____

Date _____ Location _____

Reason of doing this:
_____
_____
_____
_____

Actions we have to take:
_____
_____
_____
_____
_____

My Experience:
_____
_____
_____
_____
_____
_____

My Bucket List Goal

Date _____ Location _____

Reason of doing this:

_____
_____
_____
_____

Actions we have to take:

_____
_____
_____
_____
_____

My Experience:

_____
_____
_____
_____
_____

My Bucket List Goal _____

_____

Date _____ Location _____

Reason of doing this:

_____
_____
_____
_____

Actions we have to take:

_____
_____
_____
_____
_____

My Experience:

_____
_____
_____
_____
_____

My Bucket List Goal _____

_____

Date _____ Location _____

Reason of doing this:

_____
_____
_____
_____

Actions we have to take:

_____
_____
_____
_____
_____

My Experience:

_____
_____
_____
_____
_____

My Bucket List Goal

Date _____ Location _____

Reason of doing this:

Actions we have to take:

My Experience:

My Bucket List Goal _____

_____

Date _____ Location _____

Reason of doing this:

_____
_____
_____
_____

Actions we have to take:

_____
_____
_____
_____
_____

My Experience:

_____
_____
_____
_____
_____

My Bucket List Goal

Date _____ Location _____

Reason of doing this:

_____
_____
_____
_____

Actions we have to take:

_____
_____
_____
_____
_____
_____

My Experience:

_____
_____
_____
_____
_____
_____

My Bucket List Goal _____

_____

Date _____ Location _____

Reason of doing this:

_____
_____
_____
_____

Actions we have to take:

_____
_____
_____
_____
_____

My Experience:

_____
_____
_____
_____
_____

My Bucket List Goal

Date .... Location ....

Reason of doing this:

....

....

....

....

Actions we have to take:

....

....

....

....

....

My Experience:

....

....

....

....

My Bucket List Goal _____

_____

Date _____ Location _____

Reason of doing this:

_____
_____
_____
_____

Actions we have to take:

_____
_____
_____
_____
_____
_____

My Experience:

_____
_____
_____
_____
_____

My Bucket List Goal _____

_____

Date _____ Location _____

Reason of doing this:

Actions we have to take:

My Experience:

My Bucket List Goal

Date _____ Location _____

Reason of doing this:

_____

_____

_____

_____

Actions we have to take:

_____

_____

_____

_____

_____

My Experience:

_____

_____

_____

_____

_____

My Bucket List Goal

Date _____ Location _____

Reason of doing this:

_____
_____
_____
_____

Actions we have to take:

_____
_____
_____
_____
_____
_____

My Experience:

_____
_____
_____
_____
_____
_____

My Bucket List Goal ....

....

Date .... Location ....

Reason of doing this:

....
....
....

Actions we have to take:

....
....
....
....
....

My Experience:

....
....
....
....

My Bucket List Goal ------------------------

Date ------------------ Location ----------------

Reason of doing this:

Actions we have to take:

My Experience:

My Bucket List Goal _____

_____

Date _____   Location _____

Reason of doing this:

_____
_____
_____
_____

Actions we have to take:

_____
_____
_____
_____
_____
_____

My Experience:

_____
_____
_____
_____
_____
_____

My Bucket List Goal

Date _____ Location _____

Reason of doing this:

_____

_____

_____

_____

Actions we have to take:

_____

_____

_____

_____

_____

My Experience:

_____

_____

_____

_____

My Bucket List Goal _____

_____

Date _____ Location _____

Reason of doing this:

_____

_____

_____

_____

Actions we have to take:

_____

_____

_____

_____

_____

My Experience:

_____

_____

_____

_____

_____

My Bucket List Goal _____

_____

Date _____ Location _____

Reason of doing this:

_____
_____
_____
_____

Actions we have to take:

_____
_____
_____
_____
_____
_____

My Experience:

_____
_____
_____
_____
_____
_____

My Bucket List Goal

Date _____ Location _____

Reason of doing this:

Actions we have to take:

My Experience:

My Bucket List Goal ----------------

Date ------------- Location -------------

Reason of doing this:

Actions we have to take:

My Experience:

My Bucket List Goal _____

_____

Date _____ Location _____

Reason of doing this:

_____
_____
_____
_____

Actions we have to take:

_____
_____
_____
_____
_____
_____

My Experience:

_____
_____
_____
_____
_____

My Bucket List Goal

Date _____ Location _____

Reason of doing this:

_____
_____
_____
_____

Actions we have to take:

_____
_____
_____
_____
_____

My Experience:

_____
_____
_____
_____
_____

My Bucket List Goal

Date _____ Location _____

Reason of doing this:

_____
_____
_____
_____

Actions we have to take:

_____
_____
_____
_____
_____

My Experience:

_____
_____
_____
_____
_____

My Bucket List Goal _____

_____

Date _____ Location _____

Reason of doing this:

_____

_____

_____

_____

Actions we have to take:

_____

_____

_____

_____

_____

_____

My Experience:

_____

_____

_____

_____

_____

My Bucket List Goal

Date _____ Location _____

Reason of doing this:

_____
_____
_____
_____

Actions we have to take:

_____
_____
_____
_____
_____
_____

My Experience:

_____
_____
_____
_____
_____

My Bucket List Goal

Date _____ Location _____

Reason of doing this:

_____
_____
_____
_____

Actions we have to take:

_____
_____
_____
_____
_____
_____

My Experience:

_____
_____
_____
_____
_____

My Bucket List Goal _____

_____

Date _____ Location _____

Reason of doing this:

_____
_____
_____
_____

Actions we have to take:

_____
_____
_____
_____
_____

My Experience:

_____
_____
_____
_____
_____

My Bucket List Goal _____

_____

Date _____   Location _____

Reason of doing this:

_____

_____

_____

_____

Actions we have to take:

_____

_____

_____

_____

_____

My Experience:

_____

_____

_____

_____

_____

My Bucket List Goal _____

_____

Date _____ Location _____

Reason of doing this:

_____
_____
_____
_____

Actions we have to take:

_____
_____
_____
_____
_____
_____

My Experience:

_____
_____
_____
_____
_____
_____

My Bucket List Goal _____

_____

Date _____ Location _____

Reason of doing this:

_____

_____

_____

_____

Actions we have to take:

_____

_____

_____

_____

_____

My Experience:

_____

_____

_____

_____

_____

My Bucket List Goal ....

Date .... Location ....

Reason of doing this:

....
....
....
....

Actions we have to take:

....
....
....
....
....

My Experience:

....
....
....
....
....

My Bucket List Goal

Date _____ Location _____

Reason of doing this:

_____
_____
_____
_____

Actions we have to take:

_____
_____
_____
_____
_____

My Experience:

_____
_____
_____
_____

My Bucket List Goal _____

_____

Date _____ Location _____

Reason of doing this:

_____

_____

_____

_____

Actions we have to take:

_____

_____

_____

_____

_____

My Experience:

_____

_____

_____

_____

_____

_____

My Bucket List Goal

Date _____ Location _____

Reason of doing this:
_____
_____
_____
_____

Actions we have to take:
_____
_____
_____
_____
_____
_____

My Experience:
_____
_____
_____
_____
_____

My Bucket List Goal

Date _____ Location _____

Reason of doing this:

_____

_____

_____

_____

Actions we have to take:

_____

_____

_____

_____

_____

_____

My Experience:

_____

_____

_____

_____

_____

_____

My Bucket List Goal _____
_____

Date _____ Location _____

Reason of doing this:
_____
_____
_____
_____

Actions we have to take:
_____
_____
_____
_____
_____
_____

My Experience:
_____
_____
_____
_____
_____

My Bucket List Goal ....

....

Date .... Location ....

Reason of doing this:
....
....
....
....

Actions we have to take:
....
....
....
....
....

My Experience:
....
....
....
....
....

My Bucket List Goal _____

_____

Date _____ Location _____

Reason of doing this:

_____
_____
_____
_____

Actions we have to take:

_____
_____
_____
_____
_____

My Experience:

_____
_____
_____
_____

My Bucket List Goal

Date _____ Location _____

Reason of doing this:

_____

_____

_____

_____

Actions we have to take:

_____

_____

_____

_____

_____

_____

My Experience:

_____

_____

_____

_____

_____

My Bucket List Goal _____

Date _____ Location _____

Reason of doing this:
_____
_____
_____
_____

Actions we have to take:
_____
_____
_____
_____
_____

My Experience:
_____
_____
_____
_____
_____

My Bucket List Goal

Date _____ Location _____

Reason of doing this:

_____
_____
_____
_____

Actions we have to take:

_____
_____
_____
_____
_____

My Experience:

_____
_____
_____
_____
_____

My Bucket List Goal _____

_____

Date _____ Location _____

Reason of doing this:

_____

_____

_____

_____

Actions we have to take:

_____

_____

_____

_____

_____

_____

My Experience:

_____

_____

_____

_____

_____

My Bucket List Goal

Date _____ Location _____

Reason of doing this:

_____
_____
_____
_____

Actions we have to take:

_____
_____
_____
_____
_____
_____

My Experience:

_____
_____
_____
_____
_____

My Bucket List Goal _____

_____

Date _____   Location _____

Reason of doing this:

_____
_____
_____
_____

Actions we have to take:

_____
_____
_____
_____
_____
_____

My Experience:

_____
_____
_____
_____
_____

My Bucket List Goal ....
....

Date .... Location ....

Reason of doing this:
- -
- -
- -
- -

Actions we have to take:
- -
- -
- -
- -
- -
- -

My Experience:
- -
- -
- -
- -
- -
- -

My Bucket List Goal _____

_____

Date _____ Location _____

Reason of doing this:

_____
_____
_____
_____

Actions we have to take:

_____
_____
_____
_____
_____
_____

My Experience:

_____
_____
_____
_____
_____

My Bucket List Goal

Date _____ Location _____

Reason of doing this:
_____
_____
_____
_____

Actions we have to take:
_____
_____
_____
_____
_____

My Experience:
_____
_____
_____
_____
_____

My Bucket List Goal

Date _____ Location _____

Reason of doing this:

Actions we have to take:

My Experience:

My Bucket List Goal _____

_____

Date _____ Location _____

Reason of doing this:

_____
_____
_____
_____

Actions we have to take:

_____
_____
_____
_____
_____
_____

My Experience:

_____
_____
_____
_____
_____

My Bucket List Goal

Date _____ Location _____

Reason of doing this:
_____
_____
_____
_____

Actions we have to take:
_____
_____
_____
_____
_____

My Experience:
_____
_____
_____
_____
_____

My Bucket List Goal

Date _____ Location _____

Reason of doing this:

_____
_____
_____
_____

Actions we have to take:

_____
_____
_____
_____
_____

My Experience:

_____
_____
_____
_____
_____
_____

My Bucket List Goal _____

_____

Date _____ Location _____

Reason of doing this:

Actions we have to take:

My Experience:

My Bucket List Goal

Date _____   Location _____

Reason of doing this:

_____

_____

_____

_____

Actions we have to take:

_____

_____

_____

_____

_____

My Experience:

_____

_____

_____

_____

_____

My Bucket List Goal ----------------------

Date ------------- Location -------------

Reason of doing this:

Actions we have to take:

My Experience:

My Bucket List Goal _____

_____

Date _____ Location _____

Reason of doing this:

_____
_____
_____
_____

Actions we have to take:

_____
_____
_____
_____
_____
_____

My Experience:

_____
_____
_____
_____
_____

My Bucket List Goal _____

_____

Date _____ Location _____

Reason of doing this:

_____
_____
_____
_____

Actions we have to take:

_____
_____
_____
_____
_____

My Experience:

_____
_____
_____
_____
_____

My Bucket List Goal _____

_____

Date _____ Location _____

Reason of doing this:

Actions we have to take:

My Experience:

My Bucket List Goal _____

Date _____ Location _____

Reason of doing this:

_____
_____
_____
_____

Actions we have to take:

_____
_____
_____
_____
_____

My Experience:

_____
_____
_____
_____
_____

My Bucket List Goal

Date _____ Location _____

Reason of doing this:

_____

_____

_____

_____

Actions we have to take:

_____

_____

_____

_____

_____

My Experience:

_____

_____

_____

_____

_____

My Bucket List Goal

Date _ _ _ _ _ _ _ Location _ _ _ _ _ _ _

Reason of doing this:

_____

_____

_____

_____

Actions we have to take:

_____

_____

_____

_____

_____

My Experience:

_____

_____

_____

_____

_____

My Bucket List Goal _____

_____

Date _____ Location _____

Reason of doing this:

- -
- -
- -
- -

Actions we have to take:

- -
- -
- -
- -
- -

My Experience:

- -
- -
- -
- -
- -

My Bucket List Goal

Date _____ Location _____

Reason of doing this:

_____
_____
_____
_____

Actions we have to take:

_____
_____
_____
_____
_____

My Experience:

_____
_____
_____
_____
_____

My Bucket List Goal ....

Date .... Location ....

Reason of doing this:

Actions we have to take:

My Experience:

My Bucket List Goal

Date _____ Location _____

Reason of doing this:

_____
_____
_____
_____

Actions we have to take:

_____
_____
_____
_____
_____

My Experience:

_____
_____
_____
_____

My Bucket List Goal _____

_____

Date _____ Location _____

Reason of doing this:

_____
_____
_____
_____

Actions we have to take:

_____
_____
_____
_____
_____

My Experience:

_____
_____
_____
_____
_____

My Bucket List Goal _____

_____

Date _____ Location _____

Reason of doing this:
_____
_____
_____
_____

Actions we have to take:
_____
_____
_____
_____
_____
_____

My Experience:
_____
_____
_____
_____

www.ingramcontent.com/pod-product-compliance
Lightning Source LLC
Chambersburg PA
CBHW020543220526
45463CB00006B/2172